Essential Oil Safety

A Handbook of Safe Aromatherapy Techniques for You and Your Family

By

Bella Sherwood

Table of Contents

Introduction

There has always been a long-standing debate regarding the use of alternative therapies as opposed to the use of conventional medicine. Proponents of the former point to the gentle effectiveness of natural treatments and the lack of serious side effects that you would find when using conventional medications.

Proponents of conventional medicines claim that natural remedies, while possibly providing some assistance, are less effective overall and may not provide the cure required. They also claim that the alternative cures merely allay the symptoms whilst not dealing with the root cause.

So, where exactly does the truth lie?

I believe that the answer lies in striking balance between the two and, to explain why, I need to give you some background into my own story. You see, I was not always as happy and healthy as I am today.

At one stage in my life, I was in chronic pain – I would wake up and my whole body would be aching – not too badly but uncomfortably enough. The pain would only increase as my day went on.

By the evening, I would battle to hold my head up unsupported as the pain across the neck and shoulders was so severe and many nights I would battle to fall asleep because the pain was so severe.

I was taking anti-inflammatories on a daily basis and was told by my doctor that there was no other solution – it was something that I would have to live with.

Fortunately for me, I was not willing to live with it so I started looking into aromatherapy as an alternative to the painkillers. Up until this point, my experience with aromatherapy was in the treatment of colds and flus or to use in body products, I had not really explored the full analgesic properties of the oils.

I am pleased to say that today my life is completely different. I no longer need to rely on painkillers every day and, while I may have the occasional muscular pain, it no longer gets to the same critical levels. I no longer accept that I have to rely on dangerous chemicals to help my life better for me and I urge you to make that decision for yourself as well.

In this book I will teach you how to use essential oils in your own home and for your own family to make everyone's life better. Essential oils can be used to treat illness and pain but, more than that, they can also be used to help build your immunity and help restore your zest for life. Don't live a second-grade life for a second longer – essential oils can help you feel young again!

Chapter 1:
Essential Oils vs Conventional Medicine

Why Essential Oils Generally Come Out Tops

Just about everyone will recognize the term "aromatherapy" in some form or another. Whether you have actually used essentials oils yourself, or have seen them dotted all over the beauty aisle in a range of different products, you will have had some exposure to these oils even if you weren't aware of it at the time.

You have probably been made aware of the health benefits of using essential oils - like using Tea Tree oil to help fight against colds and flu - but were you aware that the various oils can be used effectively as beauty treatments as well?

Tea Tree oil, for example, is also a great skin treatment and can clear up acne and cuts and scratches. Palmarosa oil is a wonderful addition to a body butter because it helps the skin to regenerate. Sandalwood oil is deeply moisturizing - the list goes on and on.

Even large commercial companies acknowledge that aromatherapy oils have some value and add these oils to their products. This would seem to be a really great idea until you look a little deeper.

First and foremost, the oils are used in such tiny concentrations that they really do not do any good anyway. Secondly, the products that they are in are likely to contain a range of synthetic chemicals and preservatives - none of which are particularly good for your health.

What you need to remember is that commercially produced products are designed with the sole intent of getting you to buy them. What that means is that they are often contain little extras that you really do not need. I will bet, for example, that you always thought that the shampoo had to lather to be effective, didn't you? Well, so does everyone and that is why ingredients are added to help the shampoo lather. In fact, it is when shampoo encounters dirty hair that it less likely to lather meaning that the more the shampoo lathers, the cleaner your hair already is.

Companies want the longest shelf-life that they can get and will add preservatives to keep their product going for longer.

In addition, they add a whole lot of other things to make their product appear to work better and smell better, leaving you with a wholly synthetic product overall. Why on earth would you want to subject yourself to that when there are a lot of better options available?

Modern aromatherapy was "rediscovered" by a Frenchman named Gattefosse. He was working in his family's perfumery lab one day when he burnt his hand quite severely. The only liquid nearby was a vat of Lavender oil and so he immediately put his hand into it.

When he realized that the burn was healing a lot faster than normal and that there was no blistering, he began to become obsessed with the healing benefits of essential oils and started more research into them.

A French woman, Marguerite Maury, developed the principles of conventional aromatherapy that we follow today - she researched effective methods of dilution and application through massage.

In the last couple of decades, there has been a resurgence in interest in natural remedies as we begin to realize that there are very real, negative long term side effects associated with synthetically-manufactured medications and products.

More and more evidence is surfacing that essential oils can be just as effective as more conventional treatments but without the negative side effects.

Why should you use aromatherapy in your day to day life? Well, the fact is that you probably already are to a small extent.

Essential oils are derived from various different parts of the plant - the petals, roots, bark, peel, fruit or resin. You may come in contact with the same essences during the course of your day - take the lemon that you use for your detox drink. It is strongly scented and just through smelling the peel, you are benefiting from the essence of the plant itself.

You are basically giving yourself an aromatherapy treatment quickly and easily so why not go the whole hog and learn a bit more about using essential oils in your beauty routine as well?

Now, obviously the essential oil of a plant is a lot more concentrated than the essence that you get out of just one piece, but the idea is still the same.

Personally, I can vouch for the efficacy of these oils – as I mentioned earlier, I was told by my doctor that I simply had to learn to live with being in pain for the rest of my life. Now, essential oils did not heal me overnight but from the first time I massaged the oils into my aching muscles I could feel that they were helping.

They warmed the area and the blood flow to it increased. I felt the muscles relaxing. The pain did not go away that same night but it did ease somewhat and I slept a whole lot better. I repeated the massage the next night, and the night after that and found that the following morning I woke without as much pain and with energy that I had not had for ages.

By the end of the week, I was completely pain free. What conventional medicine couldn't do in years, aromatherapy accomplished in just under a week.

I don't bother with the aromatherapy massages every night anymore and I have found that they are not really necessary. I do still get the occasional twinge but I find that as long as I act on it fast enough, it does not escalate into something that is unmanageable. I don't even keep anti-inflammatories in the house anymore.

Are essential oils a cure-all that will work for every condition? No, they are not. Can you toss out all your prescribed medication? No, not yet. However, by applying the aromatherapy principles you will be able to improve your quality of life and possibly be able to reduce your reliance on medications going forward.

Why do aromatherapy oils come out on tops?

They are natural – Mother Nature's very own cure.

They are inexpensive – They may seem expensive when starting out but you use such small dilutions that the bottles will last you a long time.

They are effective – you will usually start to see benefits straight away.

Chapter 2:

What Other Aromatherapy Books Won't Tell You

Nature Does Deserve Respect

If I was like every other aromatherapy author out there, I would launch into how aromatherapy oils are the perfect natural cure and how you can chuck out your conventional medicine.

I am not going to advise you to chuck out your medicine. Aromatherapy can go a long way towards helping you to regain your health and vitality but there are things that it cannot do.

I don't keep anti-inflammatories in the house anymore but there are times when I will take a headache pill. Sometimes, aromatherapy is not a practical option for you. (Like when you don't want to walk into a meeting with oil all over your face.)

Sometimes you want more immediate results and, at these times, it may be more convenient to turn to conventional medicine.

I feel that, as long as it is the exception rather than the rule, there is a place for conventional medicine in your life.

If, on the other hand, you are in a situation like I was in – looking at taking pain killers every day for the rest of your life, then clearly conventional medicine is failing you and you need to look for an alternative answer.

Aromatherapy is Natural but Potent

Aromatherapy is an all-natural therapy that has got some drawbacks. Just like with conventional medicine, there are contraindications to some oils - for example, Rosemary oil, if used during pregnancy, can cause you to miscarry. Hops oil can heighten the symptoms of depression. Combining Sage oil with regular drinking can cause a toxic overload in the system.

When people look at aromatherapy oils, they tend to look at them as a natural, safe cure, something akin to herbal teas. The problem with this outlook is that it is thus more open for abuse. Whilst the oils are generally safe to use, they must be used in the correct proportions and dilutions. Unlike herbal teas, they are the highly concentrated essences of the plants themselves and so need to be treated with respect.

Did you know, for example, that you should never apply oils neat to the skin or you will risk burning the skin? (The two exceptions are Tea Tree oil and Lavender oil.) Even Chamomile oil, gentle enough to use with young children, must be diluted before being applied directly to the skin.

Taken internally, these oils can even kill you so they are not to be trifled with.

Essential Oils Can Have Side Effects

Though side effects from using essential oils tend to be mild, they can occur. Some oils like Peppermint, for example, can irritate the skin. Some oils, like Bergamot, for example, can react with sunlight and cause the skin to darken or become irritated.

Fortunately there is not a lot in terms of downsides when it comes to using essential oils, as long as you are careful about how and where you use them.

Always research the oils that you are considering using and you will be able to see whether or not they are contraindicated for you. If they are, it is no big deal, you simply have to find a different oil to use.

Chapter 3:
The Rules for Safely Using Essential Oils

Benefit and Keep Your Family Safe at the Same Time

First and foremost, let us get the safety aspects out of the way. Essential oils are natural but you do have to take some basic precautions in order to be able to use them safely and effectively.

The oils themselves are the distilled, highly concentrated compounds of the plants that they are derived from, in liquid form and this is what makes them so powerful but it is also why we need to be a bit more careful in how we apply them.

The concentrated format of the oils means that they are hundreds or thousands of times more powerful than the compounds found in nature. This makes sense because of the vast amounts of plant matter that need to be processed in order to produce just one small bottle of essential oils. That one bottle of oil contains the healing power of all the hundreds or thousands of petals/ leaves/ roots that went into the making of the oil.

Quality, Therapeutic Grade Oils

There are a lot of commercial products on the market that purport to contain essential oils. They probably do but the concentrations of essential oils in bath oils, shampoos, etc. is negligible and not likely to do you any good at all. These products may smell nice but this is not what I mean when I say that you need to incorporate essential oils into your life. You need to find 100% pure essential oils. This may mean going to a specialist store, health store or possibly searching online for the right product. In the end, the extra effort will be well worth it at the end of the day.

There are a range of products in the same aisle as the essential oils in the store. It is important to get the purest grade that you can afford - in fact, it is better to not buy any oils at all than to settle for second-grade, adulterated oils. It is also important to choose a company that has a proven track record and that will not try to pull the wool over your eyes when it comes to the oils that they sell.

The oils should say, "Therapeutic Grade" or "100% Pure". The oil should also list both the common name and the botanical name. Good companies also list how the product was distilled and which region it originally came from.

Where the Oil is From

Believe it or not, there can be a difference in the components in the oils that is region-specific. Lavender that is grown in France, for example, can be very different to that grown in the United States, even if they are the exact same species. The soil the plant is grown in, the local weather conditions and even the way it has been stored all influence the components in the oil that is eventually distilled. These components can even vary in the same field of plants from year to year. That said, don't get too bogged down by this - choose a reputable company to deal with and you can be assured that you do get what you are paying for.

How the Oils are Extracted

The process by which the oils are extracted is also important. Oils may be extracted through the use of solvents - this is usually the case with resinous oils and oils that would be damaged due to high heat due to distillation - and this is the least expensive means of extraction. The problem is that the cheaper brands of oils are generally going to contain a higher residue of these solvents.

Water or steam distillation is a more common means of extraction for higher quality oils and is used in 90% of cases. Two examples of oils that have to be extracted using solvents are Jasmine and Benzoin oil. They would not survive the distillation process.

Blends and Fragrance Oils

Words to watch out for are "Blend" or "Fragrance Oil". In the first case, the company should list exactly what oils have been used to bolster the blend. If they are honest about this, you might still be able to use the oil - just check that the oils blended in are also suitable for use on babies and kids.

Blending pure oils with less expensive ones that have similar properties or fragrance is common practice. Rose essential oil is often blended with Geranium essential oil, for example. The reason for this is that Rose absolute is ridiculously expensive to produce and most people would not be able to afford to use the absolute anyway. This need not be an issue, as long as the company does this openly. The problem comes in when you get a less scrupulous company that makes no mention that the oil has been adulterated.

You Get What You Pay For

Price is pretty much your best indication of this sharp practice. These company's usually charge a fair amount less for their oils and may even charge the same price for every oil in the range. If the price seems too good to be true, it probably is. If the prices across the range of oils for one company seem about the same, you should avoid that brand - essential oils should vary in price according to how easily they are distilled, how much plant material is used, and how common the plant is, they should never be all that same price.

Never Use Fragrance Oils - Ever

Step away from the Fragrance oils, these should never enter your home. They may smell similar to the oils but they have been synthetically produced and so have no medicinal properties whatsoever. These oils are really a cheap substitute (and here I use the word "substitute" very lightly because they really are completely different from pure essential oils. They are generally made up using cheap solvents and chemicals so I keep them far away from my kids. They should certainly never be applied to the skin - they will definitely irritate the skin and I personally don't think that they should even be inhaled. Who knows what chemicals they use?

Dilution is Essential

It is because of this high concentration of compounds that you should dilute the oils before applying them to the skin. And this applies to all essential oils, even Tea Tree oil and Lavender oil. Tea Tree oil and Lavender oil are a lot gentler on the skin and are technically gentle enough to be used neat, but may cause sensitization, especially when used on children and especially when it comes to broken skin.

To be on the safe side, I simply hardly ever use essential oils unless they have been diluted first - whether I am applying them directly to the skin or putting them in the bath water. At best, neat oils might cause irritation, at worst, they might burn the skin. In the next chapter, I will deal with exactly how best to dilute the oils for safety.

Many books will say that you can apply neat Tea Tree oil or Lavender oil to scratches, bites, etc. When it comes to babies and toddlers under the age of 6 months, this is definitely not something to take a chance with. The oils are very powerful, even when diluted, so they will still have a strong healing effect even when applied in a carrier oil.

I suggest making up a bottle of Tea Tree oil blend and a bottle of Lavender oil blend and keeping them on hand so that they are ready for use when you need them to be.

Keep Out of the Reach of Little Fingers

I learned this the hard way when my oldest son was about two years old. Like all my kids, he was a real little monkey and managed to clamber up onto the Welsh dresser to get at my bottles of essential oils. It never once occurred to me that he would clamber up. (Though looking back on it now, he was a really clever little kid and got himself into loads of sticky situations.)

He managed to open the Juniper oil (kids learn quickly and a bottle is there to be opened, as far as they are concerned - never be complacent and think that anything is safe from a kid) and slapped drops of it onto his face. He had applied about a quarter bottle before it started to sting. Fortunately I got to him quickly and wiped his face down before it got a chance to burn but his cheeks were quite red and I learned a valuable lesson - keep the oils where the kids cannot possibly get to them. I just count my lucky stars that he didn't get it into his head to drink the oils and that, because of the dropper, they only came out a little at a time. Since that time, I lock all my essential oils away.

Should the same thing happen to you, take a wet facecloth and wipe away the oils - don't forget to wipe any residue off their fingers as well - and then apply plain aqueous cream. This will help to both dilute any oils that were absorbed and soothe the stinging.

If the child gets any oils in the eyes or their mouth, your best bet is to wash the areas with milk first. The essential oils are not soluble in water and so will not be absorbed by it when it comes to the mucous membranes of the mouth or the sensitive cornea of the eye. They are, however, soluble in milk so the milk is the better option to clean out some of the essential oils. Afterwards, you can rinse with tepid water.

If the skin or eyes are burned, get the child to the emergency room as quickly as possible and be sure to tell them what oils the child used.

Taking the Oils Internally

There are people out there that advocate adding the oils to your daily diet. This is irresponsible advice at best and can actually be quite dangerous. The oils can be toxic if taken internally, even in small doses. If you suspect that your child has swallowed even a few milliliters of these oils, try and force them to vomit and get them to the doctor as quickly as possible. As little as 4ml of Eucalyptus oil, for example, can be a lethal dose.

The confusion actually came about because in French aromatherapy there is a place for the internal use of oils. It is a valid form of French aromatherapy. What should be remembered, however, is that this takes place under the supervision of a highly trained and qualified aromatherapist. For the amateur at home, it is too dangerous to take any risks and the potential rewards are simply not worth the risk.

The oils are absorbed through the skin and through inhalation a lot more quickly than would be the case if they had to work their way through your digestive system first.

NOT for Newborns

It is not advisable to start using essential oils on your baby before they are 10 weeks old. This is because their immune systems are still developing and introducing the oils at this stage could cause them to develop allergies. After they are 10 weeks old, you can start introducing the more gentle oils, such as Lavender and Chamomile.

When you do start to introduce the oils, even after the baby is 10 weeks old, you still need to check that there are no adverse reactions to the oils. Doing a patch test on the skin first and waiting for at least 12 hours to see whether or not there are any adverse reactions is really important.

If you are unsure of whether or not the oil is going to irritate the skin or not, rather diffuse a small amount of the oil in the baby's general vicinity. This can be as powerful as applying the oils to the skin, without risking irritating the baby's sensitive skin.

Again, when diffusing the oils for the first few times, watch your baby to see whether or not there are any adverse reactions - if you see signs that they are in distress or battling to breathe, get them away from the area immediately.

The Dosage Must be Right

Your child's age and size need to be taken into consideration when deciding on the appropriate dose. In general, the smaller the child, the lower the dose. Think about it for a second - your child's body is a lot smaller than yours - you would never give them the same dose of medicine as what you would personally take.

Keep in mind that every drop of oil that you add increases the concentration. I often find that people think in terms of, 1 drop per 10ml but then add in three different oils, without making the connection that this effectively increases the concentration threefold, even though you only use a single drop of each oil.

The same principle applies when it comes to essential oils as well. I will discuss the proper dosages within each age group more fully in the next chapter.

Photo-Toxic Oils

Some oils, particularly citrus oils, are photo-toxic. This is not as bad as it sounds, all it means is that the oils will react to the sun or UV light and that this can sensitize the skin, cause discoloration or a rash. When using these oils, make sure that your child will not be going out into the direct sunlight for at least an hour or two after you apply the oils. For safety sake, I reserve these oils for use in the early evening.

Store Carefully

To get the best benefits from your essential oils, you need to ensure that they are stored away from light at a fairly even, cool temperature. The same applies to the carrier oils that you will be using so it does make good sense to find a space for them in the cupboard under the stairs or in the basement. The bathroom seems like a logical space to keep the oils but, due to the amount of steam and moisture, it really is not.

Wherever you decide to store them, keep them under lock and key, especially if you have curious kids or kids that are able to walk. (Remember the lesson I learned and learn from that.)

After use be sure to close all bottles tightly to avoid the loss of oils through evaporation.

Beware of Rancid Oils

Whilst essential oils are not technically oils, they can go off after a while. Their useful lifespan will depend on the oil itself, the quality of the oil and how well they have been stored. Citrus oils, for example, tend to lose effectiveness much faster than the others and are a lot more sensitive to light and oxidation. You are typically looking at around 6 month to a couple of years. It makes sense for you to really only buy the oils that you need as you find that you need them.

Carrier oils also have a sell-by date, again, around 6 months to a couple of years and, again, depending on the type of oil, the quality of the oil and how well it has been stored. Avoid buying large quantities of carrier oils unless you are sure that you will be able to use them before they turn rancid.

The same can be said of blends. Adding a fixative oil, such as Sandalwood or Cedar Wood, for example, can extend the useful lifespan of a blend of oils and help to stabilize more volatile oils but even this will only go so far.

With both essential oils and carrier oils, changes in smell, color and texture are indicative that the oil is past its expiry date and should be thrown out. Using rancid oils will end up being a waste of time at best and can cause irritation or sensitization at best so don't take a chance - if in doubt, throw it out.

Keep it Simple

You might be keen to try and blend several oils together to get the benefits of all of them. As long as the oils all blend together well, this will not be an issue. If they are not compatible with one another, they will actually work against one another making the blend ineffective. You will normally be able to tell if a blend is bad by the way it smells - when the wrong oils are mixed together the blend will normally smell bland at best and awful at worst.

When using oils with your children, only use one oil at a time, at least to start off with. If you throw together a blend of three oils, for example, and your child has an adverse reaction, you won't know which of the oils caused the problem. Start out by using each oil on its own, separately. That way you will be able to tell whether or not the oil is going to cause sensitization or other issues. Work slowly, one oil at a time and you will soon have a few different oils that you know for a fact will cause no adverse reactions with your kids.

When you have established the oils that are safe for your kids, you can start to look at mixing different oils together. I haven't really dealt with which oils match together in this book too much but, if it is something that really interests you, there is plenty of good information out there. I would also advise investing in a directory of essential oils if this field really interests you so that you can see what oils are good for your own personal use as well.

To start off with, you can use the blends in this book as a guide - they have all been designed to be synergistic. You will quickly learn to tell good blends from bad and will eventually be able to be guided by your instincts.

In the meantime, a good general rule is to stick to oils within the same family when blending. Spice oils and citrus oils tend to blend well, as do citrus oils and wood oils. There are thousands of possible blends so I recommend blending no more than two oils together when starting out. Even now, I seldom blend more than three oils at time and I use 5 at the very most and only in special circumstances.

Oils with completely opposite beneficial properties are also not likely to make a great mix - you wouldn't want to mix an oil that stimulates the mind with one that is sedating, for example.

Keep a Record - Your Own Blend Bible

I always keep a record of every new blend that I have made. I note down what I like about the blend and what I don't like. I also note what my kid's reactions are and what actual effect the oils are having.

I have learned over the years that it is better to write down your recipes as you are making them. It only takes a few seconds extra but can save you hours of extra effort in the long-term. I still have the "Blend Bible" that I started around about 20 years ago - granted it is looking a little the worse for wear now - but it has proved invaluable in recreating blends that I found were effective.

In my case, I also had to record blends that I had made up for friends of mine - often I would get a request for a refill a few months down the line and, without my "Blend Bible" I would never have been able to keep all the different blends straight.

You are probably going to make up a few blends and tweak them as you go along. Believe me when I say that you are not going to be able to remember all the oils and quantities for all the blends that you will make. Write it all down so that, if you need to recreate a blend that worked well, you are easily able to. There really is nothing as frustrating as finding the perfect blend that works for you and forgetting what you had put into it.

Getting Blending Right

When trying a new blend, us no more than 10ml-20ml of your chosen carrier oil. That way, you won't worry about wasting ingredients. This is important because blending is largely a matter of personal taste.

Choose two to three essential oils and add them in one drop at a time, smelling the blend after each addition. This may seem painstaking at first but once you have the blend right, it will be worth it.

If one of the oils that you are using seems to be overpowering the others, add more of the lighter oils to compensate. Sandalwood, for example, is a very fragrant oil. When mixing it in a blend, I will often use it as a base and use only one part Sandalwood for every two parts of the other oils.

Do take notes and watch the concentration of the oils - add more carrier oil as needed, it won't affect the scent much at all.

Hit the Right Notes

Of course, getting the blend right means that it will smell a whole lot better. The perfume industry has this down to a fine art and you can take a note or two from their book.

A cologne or perfume hardly ever smells exactly the same on two different people because of different body chemistry. The scent also smells different over time once applied. At first, you get the heady blend of aroma, this settles down to a fuller aroma over time and finally the scent settles to its base notes.

The secret to a good blend is to blend a more volatile oil, such as Jasmine, with an oils that has a little more staying power, such as Neroli and then to finally add an oil that acts as a fixative for both, like Sandalwood. In this case, Jasmine is the top note, the fragrance that is initially smelt and quickly dissipates. Neroli is the scent that forms the bulk of the blend or the middle note and Sandalwood is the lingering fragrance or base note.

Label Everything

I also suggest labelling the jars - all you need to do is to write which oils you used and the number of drops of each oil. If you want, you can assign a number to the blend in the book or a special name for each blend and cross reference it to the book when you need to but I find that it is usually just quicker to write out the label. At the very least, record what the blend is for on the label.

Cover the label with an adhesive plastic or cello tape so that it is completely protected from cream/ oil spills. (If you don't, the label may become unreadable over time)

Don't skip this step, it really doesn't take long and you will kick yourself for not doing it when faced with a half-full bottle of oils that you cannot identify - you will not always be able to identify the blend through scent alone. I have thrown out many a half-filled bottle of oils because I couldn't remember what was in them and didn't want to risk using the wrong oils.

Patch Tests

When trying out a new blend for your child, do a patch test on your skin first. If it irritates your skin, you need to dilute the blend further and try again. Your child's skin is bound to be more sensitive than yours so if it is irritating to your skin, it is bound to be worse for your child. When you are happy that the blend is non-irritant, apply the precautions when applying the blend to your child. Do a patch test and wait at least 6-12 hours to see whether the skin reacts badly.

Do this whenever you try a completely new oil or a new blend. Also do it when you get in a new batch of oils, even if they have been fine previously and when you have made any batch of oils from scratch. It pays to also be careful with oils/blends that have been sitting at the back of the cupboard for a while - they might have gone off since you last used them.

Glass is Better

You can buy glass jars and bottles quite inexpensively from the Dollar Store so I suggest buying a few and keeping them on hand for making up your blends. Get some labels at the same time. Glass is better than plastic because the essential oils can degrade the plastic and cause chemicals from the plastic to leach into the bottle.

You can also recycle old glass jars - I find that baby food jars are particularly good. You just need to ensure that there is no lingering smell of food in the jar or in its lid. If there is, use something else as this could affect the scent of your blend.

If you are making up a blend for a once-off use, plastic is okay. If you are making a blend for longer term use, glass is far better.

Glass bottles can also be washed, sterilized and re-used. (Although they should never be used for food purposes if they have contained essential oils.) Plastic containers will need to be thrown away.

Choose bottles with tight fitting lids and choose bottles suited to your purpose. Get a bottle with a wide enough neck to make it easy to decant your carrier oils into. If you are going to be using an aqueous cream as a base, a short, wide-mouthed jar will be more useful than a bottle - when decanting and using the blend.

Start with the Lowest Concentration

When choosing essential oils, it may be tempting to add in higher concentration of oils to make the blend stronger. This is completely unnecessary and can cause irritation.

Always adhere to the guidelines laid out in Chapter 3 for safety sake. Increasing the concentration of oils will often do more harm than good - you risk damaging the health of your child if you exceed the recommended maximum concentrations of oils, especially if you do this over a prolonged period of time.

Even one dose that is too high can cause sensitization to that particular oil for life. It is far better to use smaller concentrations at first. You will be pleasantly surprised at how effective this can be.

Chapter 4:

When Aromatherapy is Not the Answer

When to Turn to More Conventional Medicine

Whilst I do advise that everyone should look to aromatherapy as an alternative therapy, I do urge caution when you are adopting the therapy if you do have health problems.

If you have serious health issues such as asthma, high blood pressure, diabetes, cancer or epilepsy or if you have to take chronic medication on a daily basis, aromatherapy may not be the answer for you right now.

I advise that you discuss the complimentary medicine with your doctor and see what their views are on it. If you want to eventually come off your medication, you will need to get their buy in to do so anyway.

In adjunct to that, I suggest that if you have serious health concerns and want to try aromatherapy, book at least one session with a qualified aromatherapist and see what they recommend. This is a far safer way to get into using essential oils and will save you the hassle, at least initially, of having to figure out which mixes work for you and which do not.

And I leave one more warning for the ladies that are pregnant. If you are in your first trimester, consider consulting a qualified aromatherapist before using essential oils. There are so many oils that can cause you to miscarry or that can raise your blood pressure and you really do not want to put baby at risk, do you?

Generally speaking, if you are unsure whether or not the oil is safe for you to use, it is best to get professional help before trying it out.

Chapter 5:
Oils That Can be Used by the Whole Family

Oils to Make Blends With

The most important thing to consider when using oils in a blend to treat stress, anxiety or depression is that the child really needs to like the oil. The right blend of oils can be like sunshine in a bottle, instantly lifting the spirits when used.

Once you have found a blend that your child really likes, it is a good idea to allow them to use it on a regular basis to help ward off depression and stress in future.

This can be done simply and effectively, without asking your child's permission by diffusing the oils into the atmosphere.

This is especially useful when you have a teenager in the house who is particularly fractious and sensitive. If tensions in the house are running high, diffusing oils into the air is a really good way to calm everyone down.

Getting your teenager involved in making their own blends and choosing the oils that suits them can help to increase their buy-in of the remedy.

The following oils are useful for calming and treating the symptoms of nervous tension, stress, insomnia: Chamomile, Bergamot, Sandalwood, Lavender, Sweet Marjoram, Lemon Balm, Valerian, and Lemon.

If your child is suffering from fatigue brought on by exam stress, these oils are helpful: Basil, Jasmine, Peppermint, Ylang Ylang, Neroli, Angelica, Rosemary.

If your child battles with their nerves, you can help them by using the following oils: Chamomile, Clary Sage, Juniper, Lavender, Marjoram, Rosemary.

If you child is battling anxiety and stress-related symptoms the following oils are useful for re-balancing the adrenal functions: Basil, Geranium, Rosemary, Clary Sage, and Pine.

There are not a lot of oils that can be used by the whole family but Lavender oil, Tea Tree oil and Chamomile oil do fall into this category. There is one caveat though - infants under the age of 10 weeks should not be exposed to any essential oils at all - their systems are not strong enough yet to handle it.

Lavender

This is the most useful oil and one that is generally liked. Whilst it is classified as a floral oil, the scent has enough of an herby twist to it to make it acceptable for use by men as well.

It is great to apply to a small scratch or cut, it helps soothe an insect bite and I have gotten rid of a lot of rashes by using Lavender oil. What I do like is that you can apply it neat. I personally do not like it for treating my headaches but my mother loves it and rubs a drop into each temple as soon as she feels one coming on.

If you do love the scent, that is great. Apply it to tight muscles, let someone who has just had a shock sniff it. Spritz it on your pillows at night to encourage a deep, restful sleep.

Tea Tree

This one has a smell that is best described as clinical and even the manliest man cannot say that it is too "girly". It is another oil that is of great use in treating cuts and scrapes and is a potent anti-bacterial and anti-fungal agent. If I cut myself, I throw on some tea tree oil and forget about it. When I am neglecting my nails, I tend to get painful hangnails and apply tea tree oil to help them heal faster.

When it comes to fighting just about any kind of bug or virus, tea tree in the diffuser will help to sanitize the air. If someone at home has flu, burn Tea Tree oil all around the house to help prevent the flu spreading to others. Apply a little to the sinuses to help kill off germs in that area.

It is a great treatment for fungal infections like ringworm and make a great tick and flea treatment for your dog. I sneak on a drop of Tea Tree oil at the base of my dog's necks and their tails and it is really effective at keeping ticks and fleas away. I am told that it will work in a similar manner with cats as well but apparently my cats never got that memo - I cannot get near them with the bottle.

Tea tree can also be applied neat - great when you are in a hurry.

Chamomile

When it comes to pain relief, chamomile is my go to oil. It cannot be applied neat so do dilute it before using. I apply it to my cheek when I have toothache and it works amazingly well.

If I have a headache, I add a few drops of chamomile to some cool water and soak a wash cloth in it. Wring out the cloth and you have a perfect compress - if the headache is really bad, I might also add a drop or two of lavender. I then make two compresses - one for the back of my neck and one to put over the eyes. Then it is off to a quiet room for a bit of a lie down - works wonders even with migraines.

Chamomile is also very soothing for the skin - rashes, especially allergic ones, respond well to it. A bonus is that it also helps the skin feel soft. It is gentle enough to be used on the face, if diluted, and also by people who have sensitive skin.

If you have bad sunburn, or wind burn, or chapped lips, mix some chamomile, lavender and sandalwood together in an aqueous base.

If you have a toddler that is prone to throwing temper tantrums, keep chamomile oil, diluted in a suitable carrier oil. I have found that rubbing this mixture on their hands and back of the neck can help to reduce the severity of the temper tantrum, sometimes even cutting it off completely.

Blends for Your Family

Oil to Help Ease Muscle Pains after the First Trimester of Pregnancy

Carrier Oils:

20ml Sweet Almond oil

Essential Oils:

3 drops Vetiver oil

3 Drops Geranium oil

3 Drops Sandalwood oil

Rub into the area at least once or twice a day.

Blend for Itchy Skin Complaints and Rashes in Young Children

1 Drop Chamomile oil

1 Drop Lavender oil

Mix into 20ml of sweet almond oil or a blend of sweet almond and avocado oils (10ml each.) Massage over the whole body, avoiding the genitals.

This blend can also help baby sleep.

Blend for Colic in Young Children

1 Drop Mandarin oil or 1 Drop Sweet Orange oil and 1 drop of Lavender oil, mixed into 20ml of a carrier oil of your choice and massaged into the back, chest and abdomen twice a day.

Sleepy Time Mix

(Suitable for ages 10 weeks and up)

1 drop Lavender oil

1 drop Chamomile oil

20ml carrier oil of your choice

Mix all ingredients and massage into back, chest and feet just before bedtime.

Anti-Stress Blend

(Suitable for ages 2 years and up)

This blend is ideal for tweens and teenagers that are stressed out because of exams.

2 drops Sandalwood oil

2 drops Ylang Ylang oil

2 drops Vetiver oil

40ml carrier oil of your choice

Mix all the ingredients together and rub into the neck and shoulders to relieve tension there. Also rub into the soles of the feet. Alternatively add the oils to the bath or a diffuser. The Vetiver and Sandalwood are deeply relaxing and the Ylang Ylang helps to lift the blend.

A drop or two of the blend rubbed into the temples is instantly calming and can help to relieve stress and tension during the day as well.

Insomnia Blend for Older Children

(Suitable for ages 6 and up)

3 drops Chamomile oil   75ml carrier oil of your choice

3 drops Ylang Ylang oil

3 drops Lavender oil

3 drops Cedar Wood oil

Blend all ingredients together and rub onto the chest and back and into the soles of the feet. It is a very soothing mix for sore muscles as well.

Spirit Lifting Oil

2 Drops Neroli oil

2 Drops Lavender oil

2 Drops Ylang Ylang oil

2 Drops Sandalwood oil

Use this in a diffuser, or add to 20ml of a carrier oil of your choice and massage into skin.

Pick-Me-Up Blend

2 Drops Neroli oil

2 Drops Benzoin oil

2 Drops Cedar Wood oil

Use this in a diffuser, or add to 20ml of a carrier oil of your choice and massage into skin. Alternatively, add it to your bath water.

Chapter 6:
Remedies Best Applied Through Diffusion

When it comes to the use of essential oils, steam treatments and vaporization are ideal ways to get the full benefit of the oils without actually coming into direct contact with them at all. This is of especial benefit when you want to help ease breathing, calm the mind and is an effective beauty treatment as well.

Diffusing Oils

This is a great way to scent the rooms of your home, without worrying about the smoky atmosphere created by incense. Oils are vaporized by heating them up and causing them to diffuse into the air in your home.

An aromatherapy burner or diffuser are ideal methods of delivery, especially if you plan to make use of the therapy often. As an alternative, and if you still use incandescent light bulbs, you can look for a ceramic ring that fits on top of the bulb. You then add a few drops of oil to the ring and it is warmed by the bulb.

If you have a radiator or use a heater or fire in winter, you can just fill a bowl with water and drop some oils into that. Keep the bowl in close proximity to the heat source and they will evaporate. Adding a bowl of water can also help to replace the humidity in a room when a heater is used.

Oils have long been used in rituals to create a specific ambience - Frankincense is traditionally used for promoting relaxation and reflectiveness of mind. Oils can also be vaporized in order to clear off unpleasant odors like cigarette smoke and oils such as Lemongrass and Citronella have a firm value when it comes to being insect repellents.

In ancient medicinal texts, the burning of Rosemary and Juniper leaves was recommended to cleanse the air and to prevent the spread of infection. Rosemary is too stimulating to use at night so you can choose Eucalyptus oil or Myrtle oil in its place in the sickroom at night. Both are very effective at clearing congestion and easing breathing.

It is important to keep any aromatherapy burners out of the reach of children and pets - dogs may lap up the water or knock over the burner causing problems. Kids may do the same.

Steam Inhalation

When you are ill and battling congestion, there is nothing better to clear out the mucous and the germs than a steam treatment. This is easily accomplished - all you need is to fill a bowl with hot water, add around about 5 drops of your chosen oil and to bend over the bowl and drape a towel over both your head and the bowl. This creates a mini-steam chamber. Inhale deeply to allow the sinuses to unblock and to ensure that the vapor is drawn deep into the body so that germs and viruses are killed.

Stay in your "steam room" for at least 5-10 minutes so that the sinuses have a good chance to clear. You can alternatively use a hot bath though the effect is not as concentrated. This treatment is not recommended if you have high blood pressure or are an epileptic.

Anti-Flu Steam Treatment

2 Drops Eucalyptus oil

2 Drops Peppermint oil

1 Drop Lavender oil

Add the oils to the steaming water and drape the towel around the head and breathe in deeply until the sinuses clear.

Cold and Cough Steam Treatment

2 Drops Juniper Berry oil

1 Drop Rosemary oil

2 Drops Lime oil

Add the oils to the steaming water and drape the towel around the head and breathe in deeply until the sinuses clear.

Cold and Flu Be-Gone

5 drops eucalyptus

5 drops tea tree oil

5 drops mandarin oil

Mix all the ingredients together and diffuse. This will help to clear out the germs from the sick room and also clear up congestion at the same time.

Cold and Flu Diffuser Blend

3 drops Tea Tree oil

3 drops Eucalyptus oil

3 drops Lavender oil

Diffuse throughout your home to kill off airborne germs and bacteria. This blend will also help to ease congestion.

Steam Treatment for a Bad Cough That Just Won't Quit

2 Drops Frankincense oil

2 drops Myrrh oil

2 Drops Bergamot oil

Add the oils to the steaming water and drape the towel around the head and breathe in deeply until the sinuses clear.

Steam Treatment for Hay Fever and Asthma

2 Drops Eucalyptus oil

2 Drops Lavender oil

Add the oils to the steaming water and drape the towel around the head and breathe in deeply until the sinuses clear. Steam treatments are great for Hay fever as they clear the passageways and can help to humidify the mucous membrane of the nose and lungs.

Steam Treatments for Beauty

Steam treatments can be helpful when it comes to unblocking your pores and livening up a dull complexion. If you have dry or sensitive skin or thread veins, you should avoid steam treatments for beauty purposes.

Basically, all you need is to fill a bowl with hot water, add around about 5 drops of your chosen oil and to bend over the bowl and drape a towel over both your head and the bowl. Steam the skin in this manner for about 5 minutes or so, once or twice a week at most. When finished, wipe the face with a wash cloth that has been soaked in warm, clean water to remove debris that has come to the surface of the skin and follow up by splashing the skin with cool water to help close the pores again. Pat skin dry and apply either Witch Hazel or Rose Water before moisturizing.

You can also find special facial saunas that make this process easier but these are not essential.

Steam Treatment for Oily Skin

2 Drops Juniper oil

2 Drops Lavender oil

Add the oils to the steaming water and drape the towel around the head. Stay in position for about 5 minutes. When finished, wipe the face with a wash cloth that has been soaked in warm, clean water to remove debris that has come to the surface of the skin and follow up by splashing the skin with cool water to help close the pores again. Pat skin dry and apply either Witch Hazel or Rose Water before moisturizing.

Steam Treatment for Cleansing Pores

2 Drops Lemon oil

2 Drops Tea Tree oil

Add the oils to the steaming water and drape the towel around the head. Stay in position for about 5 minutes. When finished, wipe the face with a wash cloth that has been soaked in warm, clean water to remove debris that has come to the surface of the skin and follow up by splashing the skin with cool water to help close the pores again. Pat skin dry and apply either Witch Hazel or Rose Water before moisturizing.

Steam Treatment for Balancing Skin

2 Drops Jasmine/ Rose oil

2 Drops Lavender oil

1 Drop Geranium oil

Add the oils to the steaming water and drape the towel around the head. Stay in position for about 5 minutes. When finished, wipe the face with a wash cloth that has been soaked in warm, clean water to remove debris that has come to the surface of the skin and follow up by splashing the skin with cool water to help close the pores again. Pat skin dry and apply either Witch Hazel or Rose Water before moisturizing.

Clear the Cobwebs Blend

2 drops Peppermint oil

2 drops Rosemary oil

Diffuse these oils in the room where your child is studying to help them focus and concentrate. These oils stimulate the mind so should not be used within a couple of hours of bedtime.

Anti-Stress Blend

3 drops Benzoin oil

3 drops Cedar Wood oil

3 drops Sweet Orange oil

This blend is best if used in a diffuser. Expose your child to it at for at least half an hour a day during high stress periods.

Anti-Stress Bottle Blend

2 drops Chamomile oil

2 drops Lavender oil

2 drops Neroli oil

You will need to get a small bottle with a tight-fitting lid. Place a clean tissue or piece of cotton rag into the bottle and add the essential oils.

Give it to your child to keep with them. They can take a whiff of the oils when they are feeling especially anxious. (It is a good idea to explain what this is all about to their teachers if they are going to be taking the bottle to school with them and using it there.)

Chapter 7:
Remedies Best Used In the Bath

Diffusion will not Always Work

The ancient Romans understood the importance of hydrotherapy. A trip to the baths was about more than just personal hygiene and could last a few hours - it was a place to relax and unwind, to discuss business and even a place to improve physical fitness.

The idea was to induce sweating by moving through a series of rooms, each one hotter than the last. Most public baths would have the same set up. You would start in an Apodyterium, the ancient equivalent of a locker room. Next up would be a visit to the Frigidarium, the cold room which had a bath of cold water. After than you would move to a Tepidarium, a room that was warmer. The final room in the series, the Caldarium was the hottest room and was always heating using a brazier. There were usually basins containing cool water to allow you to cool off in need.

You would generally round everything off by having a massage using essential oils. The oils would be scraped off and you would either proceed to the Laconium to rest, if there was one, or back to the Apodyterium to get dressed and be on your way.

These ancient baths formed the basis for what we would now call a modern spa and the treatment potential is just as important now as it was back then.

Whilst today we may not have the time to spend the whole morning in the bath, a quick session in the sauna can produce benefits as well. For those who have no access to a sauna, a bath or shower will do just as well. Cranking up the hot water in the bath or shower and letting the steam clear your senses is as therapeutic as sitting in a sauna.

Essential Oils in the Bath

Essential oils can help you elevate the treatment potential of your bath exponentially. And it is so easy - simply draw your bath and add in a few drops of the essential oils of your choice just before you climb in. It really couldn't be simpler.

The oils themselves will not diffuse in the water but the heat from the water will help the oils to evaporate - that is why you should only add them after the bath has been drawn.

It is important to add, at the very most, 6 drops of essential oils in a full bath because of the potential to irritate the skin. What I advise is to start with no more than two drops of one particular oil and to note the reaction to your skin. Add another oil in a different session and you will quickly find which oils irritate the skin and which do not.

The key to avoiding irritation is to be careful about the number of oils added - bath time is not the time to try complex blends and to limit your bath to no longer than 20 or 30 minutes at most. Irritation does not necessarily mean that you will develop a rash - your skin may become red, tingly or intensely itchy. If this happens, get out of the bath, dry yourself off and apply an aqueous cream to the affected areas.

I usually find though that simply drying myself off is often enough to get rid of any irritation.

Cold & Flu Fighting

2 Drops Eucalyptus oil

2 Drops Juniper oil

2 Drops Sweet Orange oil

2 Cups Epsom salts (Optional)

½ Cup Baking soda (Optional)

The Epsom salts and baking soda should be left out if you have high blood pressure or are pregnant.

Run a hot bath, adding the Epsom salts and Baking soda while drawing the bath so that they dissolve. Just before climbing into the bath, add your oils. Relax for at least 20 minutes. Dry yourself off and wrap up warmly when you are finished in the bath. This bath will detox your system and cause you to sweat the virus out.

Restore the Skin's pH Balance

2 Drops Geranium oil

2 Drops Sandalwood oil

1 cup Apple Cider Vinegar

Draw a tepid bath. Mix the oils with the Apple Cider vinegar and add to the bath just before you climb in. Soak for at least 20 minutes.

A Bath for Emotional Balance

2 Drops Sweet Orange oil

2 Drops Jasmine oil

2 Drops Sandalwood chips

When everything seems just a bit too overwhelming, a bath can be extremely good medicine. Just add to the bath after the water has drawn and relax with a glass of good wine and a good book. You'll literally be able to feel the tension draining away.

A Sleep Inducing Bath

2 Drops Chamomile oil

2 Drops Lemon Balm oil

2 Drops Valerian oil

Draw a fairly warm bath around about an hour before you want to go to sleep and add the oils once the bath is drawn. If you want to really increase the detoxification power and increase relaxation, also add a cup of Epsom salts. Relax in the bath for about 20 minutes. When you get out, you should feel completely relaxed and almost ready for bed.

Happiness Bath

1 Tablespoon of Sweet Almond oil

4 Drops of Marjoram oil

4 Drops of Clary Sage oil

4 Drops of Rosemary or Cypress oil

2 Drops Hyssop oil

1 Drop Lemon Balm oil

This is a great bath mixture for when you have had a bad day at work but still need to put in a shift at home. This bath is best taken in the early evening because the Rosemary oil or Cypress oil can stimulate the mind.

Mix all the oils together and then draw your bath. A tepid bath rather than hot bath is better. Add the oils just before you climb into it.

Anti-Cellulite Treatment

1 cup Epsom salts

½ cup Rock Salt

Add 8-10 drops of the following blend of oil to the salt:

8 Drops of Basil oil

14 Drops of Grapefruit oil

6 Drops of Juniper oil

12 Drops of Lemon oil

6 Drops of Oregano oil

2 Tablespoons olive oil

Blend together well and use as a scrub for affected areas. Leave on for a few minutes and then climb into the bath and soak for about 20 minutes.

Alternatively, switch out the rock salt for coffee grinds and do the same, except this time instead of climbing into the bath, rinse off in the shower.

Milk and Honey Bath

This recipe does sound messy but it really is wonderful for your skin and well worth trying when your skin is tired and dry.

4 Tablespoons Honey

6 Tablespoons Dried Milk Powder blended with enough boiling water to form a paste

1 cup of boiling water

5 Drops Sandalwood oil

5 Drops Jasmine oil

5 Drops Rose oil

Mix the honey into the water and then add the milk powder paste and blend until the honey has dissolved and all lumps in the milk powder have been removed. While you are drawing your bath, add in the milk powder/ honey water under the running taps so that it dissolved properly.

When the water is just ready for you to climb in, add the essential oils and relax.

Milky Skin Softening Bath

2 Cups Dried Full-Fat Powdered Milk

1/2 Cup Epsom salts

1/2 Cup Baking soda

6 Drops Sandalwood oil

5 Drops Benzoin oil

4 Drops Neroli oil

Draw a bath and add the powdered ingredients to it under the running water so that it dissolved properly.

When the water is just ready for you to climb in, add the essential oils and relax.

Oatmeal Milk Bath

¼ Cup Oatmeal

½ Cup Dried Powdered Milk

1 Tablespoon Hazelnut oil

6 drops Lavender oil

Put oats in muslin bag, tie it shut and throw in while the water is running. When you have soaked a little, use the muslin bag as a sponge to get all the goodness out of the oats. Add the powdered milk to the bath under the running water so that it dissolves properly.

When the water is just ready for you to climb in, add the essential oils and relax.

Soothing Skin Soak

4 Cups Dried Powdered Milk mixed into enough boiling water to form a smooth paste

2 Chamomile Tea Bags

5 Drops Chamomile oil

5 Drops Lavender oil

1 Teaspoon Calendula oil

Draw a bath and add the powdered milk to it under the running water so that it dissolves properly. Drop the tea bags in at the same time. Mix all the oils together.

When the water is just ready for you to climb in, add the essential oils and relax.

Add the Oils to Some Full-Fat Milk

Oils will not diffuse in water but the fat in the milk helps them to do just that. Use about a cup of milk and, again, no more than 6 drops of essential oil. Mix the two together and then add to the bath just before getting in. Swirl the water to mix in the milk.

This has the added benefit of being good for your skin as well. It is said that Cleopatra used to bath in asses' milk to keep her skin young and supple and modern research shows that there may be some truth in that - the lactic acid in the milk can help to slough off dead skin cells and so help to soften skin.

Beauty Bath Fit for a Queen (or King)

2 Drops Sandalwood oil

2 Drops Ylang Ylang oil

2 Drops Neroli oil

1 Cup Full-fat milk

Draw a tepid bath - in this case the bath water should not be too hot. Mix the essential oils into your milk. Just before you get into the bath, add the milk mixture and swirl the water so that it is properly incorporated. Relax for about 20 minutes.

Itchy Skin Relief

2 Drops Lavender oil

2 Drops Geranium oil

2 Drops Palmarosa oil

1 Cup oatmeal

1 Cup milk

A few sprigs Lavender flowers (if you have them in the garden)

A muslin bag

Place the oatmeal in the muslin bag and hang it under the hot tap as you are drawing your bath. The bath water should be tepid rather than hot. Once the bath has been drawn, toss the oatmeal bag into it. Mix the oils and the milk and then add to the bath just before climbing into it.

Use the muslin bag with the oatmeal in it as a sponge, concentrating on the itchy areas.

Add the Oils to Your Body First

Another option is to blend your chosen oils into a carrier oil and to massage them into your skin before you get into the bath. I find that this is particularly effective when it comes to relieving muscular aches and pains and is a great way to reduce skin irritation.

For full benefits, massage the blend into the areas as necessary and allow to settle for at least 15-20 minutes before climbing into a bath that is as warm as you can manage. The heat of the water helps to further increase the absorption of any excess oils and also helps to relieve soreness as well.

Athlete's Rub

3 Drops Rosemary oil

2 Drops Lemon Grass oil

50ml Jojoba oil

Mix oils into oil, ensuring that they are well incorporated. Massage into sore muscles and leave in place for at least 20 minutes.

Draw a hot bath and soak for at least 20 minutes.

Chronic Pain Reliever

 2 Drops Melissa oil

2 Drops Sweet Marjoram oil

2 Drops Chamomile oil

10ml Carrier oil of your choice

10ml Jojoba oil

Blend all ingredients together and massage into affected areas twice daily or as needed.

You can also cut out the carrier oil and Jojoba oil and use these oils in a hot bath instead. If you are not epileptic and do not have high blood pressure, you can also add 2 cups of Epsom Salts to the bath to help relieve pain.

Using a Foot Bath

Perhaps you do not have a bath in your home, or perhaps you simply do not want to go to all the trouble of drawing one. A foot bath can be an effective alternative, especially when it comes to relieving the symptoms of colds and the flu.

Simply select a basin that is big enough to accommodate both feet and half-fill with warm water.

Add in the oils of your choice and soak your feet for at least 15-20 minutes.

Fast Fix for Fatigued Feet

I use this remedy of I have had to stand for long periods of time and I find that it is particularly effective for sore feet.

You will need:

A basin big enough to fit your feet in

2 Golf balls

1 Drop Lavender oil

1 Drop Eucalyptus oil

1 Drop Peppermint oil

Half-fill the basin with water as hot as you can manage. Place the golf balls into the basin as well and then add in the oils. Soak your feet in the water, every now and again rolling your soles over the golf balls - this helps to relieve muscular tension in the feet.

Soak for about 20 minutes and then wrap them with a towel, elevate your feet and rest with feet elevated for about 20 minutes. Apply a rich aqueous cream to which you have added some Lavender oil and socks and leave on for at least 20 minutes or, if possible, overnight.

Hydrotherapy Made Easy

One of the most effective treatments when it comes to boosting circulation is to use hot and cold water alternatively. There are a couple of ways that you can do this at home - either in the shower or in the bath.

In the Shower

After your normal shower, turn the tap to as cold as you can manage for about 2 minutes and then switch back to warm water again for about two minutes. Repeat a couple of times. This is a great way to boost circulation, rev up the metabolism, wake you up and firm up the skin in the areas concerned. Always end on a warm note.

Power Shower

2 Drops Peppermint oil

2 Drops Rosemary oil

1 Clean wash cloth

Dampen the wash cloth and add the oils to it. Turn on the shower and place the wash cloth at your feet. The heat of the shower will release the scent of the oils and you will feel invigorated. Finish off with blasts of cold and warm water to really wake you up.

Breast Firming Shower

2 Drops Neroli oil

2 Drops Rose oil blend

2 Drops Jasmine oil blend

60ml Rose Hip oil

This time we are not going to use the oils until after your shower. Alternate hot and cold water, concentrating on the breast area. Climb out of the shower and dry the skin on the breasts and décolletage. Apply the Rose Hip oil and essential oil blend and leave to soak in while you dry the rest of your body. Mop up any excess oil with a clean wash cloth or tissue.

Sitz Bath

Whilst the ancient Romans had the luxury of being able to plunge into a cool bath of water after being in very hot room, most of us cannot boast the same luxury. A sitz bath is a good alternative and can be very effective but it is not suitable if you have high blood pressure or suffer from epilepsy.

You will need two basins large enough to sit in. Half fill one basin with very warm water and the other basin with very cold water. The idea is to sit in one basin and then put your feet in the other basin and stay this way for about 5 minutes before switching. Do this at least twice. Be warned, this is not for the faint-hearted - that cold basin will be a shock to the system, but that is the whole point, after all.

It is a good way to boost immunity, boost circulation and improve lymph drainage so it is worth persevering.

Anti-Thrush/ Cystitis Sitz Bath

2 Drops Bergamot oil

2 Drops Sandalwood oil

Place oils in warm bath just before climbing into it. Soak for five minutes before switching baths. Repeat at least twice.

Chapter 8:
Remedies Best Used Applied to the Skin and Hair

When Only Application is Going to Work

There are times when you need to apply the essential oils to your skin or muscles to get the full effect. For cosmetic purposes, adding the oils into the bath or steaming your face with them will only go so far. You do need to capitalize on the overall effect by adding essential oils to your body cream or moisturizing lotion.

There are also times medicinally when only application to the skin or hair will work. For example, if you have ring worm, joint pain or dirty hair, vaporization of the oils will not do you all that much good.

In this chapter we will go through treatments that need to be applied to the skin or hair and will deal with products on both the medicinal and cosmetic sides of the scale.

The following two creams are very nourishing for your skin, will boost moisture and reduce the appearance of fine lines and wrinkles and help to reverse sun damage and scarring.

Super Smooth Night Cream

100ml Rose Hip oil

10ml Avocado oil

5 Drops Sandalwood oil

5 Drops Geranium oil

5 Drops Neroli oil

5 Drops Rose oil

5 Drops Lavender oil

Clean and tone face as you normally would. Using your ring finger, put a dot of oil onto each cheekbone and then pat it in until absorbed across the whole cheek. A patting motion may take a little longer but it is less likely to cause the dragging of your skin that can lead to wrinkling and it helps to boost circulation to the skin as well.

Use another two of these drops to cover your forehead and temples. One more dot should be enough to cover the T-Zone. Avoid the eye area with this oil. You'll need about three dots for the neck and about four for the décolletage. Finish off by dotting one dot onto the back of each hand and massaging in. (The hand are just as important when it comes to beating the signs of aging but are more likely to show signs of neglect.)

Relax for 5-10 minutes, placing a warmed wash cloth - damp not soaking - over the face to further assist the absorption of the oils. Dab off any excess after this time and pat skin dry.

This starts working to clarify and moisturize your skin from the very first treatment.

Daily Beauty Cream

Naturally, you want different things from your night and day cream!

80 ml aqueous cream, preferably organic

5 Drops Geranium oil

10 Drops Palmarosa oil

5 Drops Sandalwood oil

Cleanse and tone skin and apply the cream. Go off to style your hair or start breakfast so that the cream is completely absorbed before applying your make up.

These two simple creams will help heal your skin and it will soon start to look younger and more refined.

The day cream is mild enough to be used by people of all skin types because Geranium oil is a skin regulator - it helps to moisturize dry skin and helps to regulate sebum production thus curbing acne as well.

Easy Face Scrub

1 Clean Wash cloth

½ Cup Oatmeal Flakes

2 Drops Lavender oil

2 Drops Neroli oil (If you have a dry skin)

2 Drops Tea Tree oil (If you have oily skin)

Place the oatmeal in the center of the wash cloth and drop the oils onto it. Scrunch the wash cloth up so that the oatmeal and oil mixture are completely enclosed. Soak in warm water for a couple of minutes and then gently massage over the skin.

The wash cloth should only be used for this purpose and should never be washed in fabric softener. That way, it will provide a good, gentle scrubbing surface. The oatmeal inside will also help to intensify the cleansing action but, with the oils, the action of the oatmeal liquid will be even better.

Honey Face Mask

10 ml Avocado oil or half a medium-sized avocado, pitted, peeled and mashed

2 Tablespoons Honey

10ml Sweet Almond oil

2 Drops Neroli oil

2 Drops Jasmine oil

2 Drops Rose oil

Mix together all ingredients and apply to face. Leave on for 20-30 minutes and then rinse of with tepid water. This is messy but highly effective for dry and mature skin.

Fruit Facials

You can also use the peels of the fruit that you eat as a supplementary beauty treatment. Rub the inside of the peel on your skin for an instant boost. Banana is very moisturizing and papaya is great for oilier skin. Leave the "treatment" on for a few minutes and rinse in tepid water.

In our house, you need to keep the skin peels out of the dog's reach - our schnauzer, Pickle, thinks that Papaya skin is a great treatment for her tummy and she loves it.

Flower Waters

Making your own flower waters at home is fairly simple. All you need to do is to mix about 20 - 30 drops of the essential oil that you choose into 100ml of distilled water.

Put this in a dark cupboard for about a week and then run it through a coffee filter to remove all traces of the oils. Although essential oils do not dissolve in water they do impart their scent to it as well as their properties.

This method can be very helpful in the prevention and treatment of skin conditions such as acne, dermatitis and eczema, and to generally tone and cleanse the complexion.

Almost any oil can be used, but the more traditional ones include rose, orange blossom, lavender and petitgrain; alternatively, blended flower waters can be made to suit specific complexions.

Orange Blossom water is probably the most famous skin treatment of all and was, according to legend, first used by the then Queen of Hungary to keep her young and beautiful. It was apparently so effective that she found a husband more than two decades her junior and she was hailed as one of the most beautiful women in history!

Using Milk as a Treatment

The lactic acid in milk acts to gently exfoliate the skin and to improve its ability to retain moisture. You can either add it to your bath water or use it as a facial cleanser - it is especially good for those with blemishes or greasy skin.

If using it in the bath, ½ to 1 cup of full-fat milk is best.

If using as a cleanser, make only enough to last the day and add 2-3 drops of your chosen essential oil for every 5 teaspoons of milk.

Goat's milk is better than cow's milk, especially in the cases where skin allergies and eczema are present but make do with whatever you have on hand.

Make Your Own Talcum or Baby Powder

You can also make use of body powder to help to scent your skin. Rice flour makes a perfect replacement for synthetic flours for yourself or your baby. The powder is fine and clear of colorants and nasty chemicals.

If using it for yourself, mix yourself the powder and make up a matching perfume for you to wear. Add a few drops to the bath and you will have a perfectly layered scent.

For every tablespoon of rice flour, you can add 1-2 drops of essential oils, depending on how heavily scented you want the mixture to be.

The powder will last well if kept in a container that seals properly and that is airtight.

Use whenever you want to for a scent boost.

Witch Hazel as a Toner

Many people with oily skins need more than just a cleanser to keep their skins under control. You will find that a mixture of Rose Water and Witch Hazel makes a nice astringent that will remove all traces of cleanser and further clarify the pores.

Mix in 50ml of Lavender oil and 50 ml of Rose Water with 2 drops of Lavender oil and 2 drops of Tea Tree oil to make an effective, but non-drying toner for skins that are combination/ normal or greasy.

If you have sensitive skin, Witch Hazel will probably be a bit too harsh for it so mix in 75ml of either Orange Water or Rose Water with 25ml Witch Hazel with 2 drops of Lavender oil and 2 drops of Neroli oil for a toner that will sooth skin without drying it out.

The Best Essential Oils for Skin Care

For skin regeneration you cannot beat Lavender oil, Chamomile oil, Rose oil, Neroli oil, Frankincense oil, Palmarosa oil and Geranium oil.

For dry skin use: Lavender oil, Chamomile oil, Rose oil, Neroli oil, Frankincense oil, Geranium oil or Sandalwood oil.

For oily skin use: Lavender oil, Tea Tree oil, Geranium oil, Juniper Berry oil, Lemon oil or Rosemary oil.

Treatments for Your Hair

The Ultimate Hair Conditioner for Oily Hair

This helps to condition the hair and to stimulate growth.

25ml Olive oil, slightly warmed.

5 Drops Rosemary oil

5 Drops Lavender oil

Add the essential oils to the warmed olive oil. Apply to the scalp, massaging in. Wrap your head in cling wrap and a warm towel. Leave on for 20 minutes before rinsing out.

The Ultimate Hair Conditioner for Dry Hair

25ml Jojoba oil, slightly warmed

5 Drops Vertiver oil

5 Drops Lavender oil

Warm the oil using the method mentioned above. Add the oils. Apply to the scalp, massaging in. Wrap your head in cling wrap and a warm towel. Leave on for 20 minutes before rinsing out.

On the Go Scalp Rub

5 Drops Lavender oil

5 Drops Tea Tree oil

Massage the oils into your scalp and carry on with your day. You do not need to rinse them out of your hair.

Hair Tonic

10 Drops Rosemary oil (if you have oily hair)

10 Drops Chamomile oil (if you have dry hair)

1 Tablespoon of Apple Cider Vinegar

50ml Rose Water

50 ml Lavender Water

Mix the ingredients together well and then massage into the scalp. Leave on for at least half an hour or, if at all possible, overnight. If you can get away with it, do not rinse out until the next time you need to wash your hair, the longer it stays on, the better.

Dry Shampoo

1 Drop Rosemary oil

1 Tablespoon Powdered Orris Root or Fuller's Earth

Mix all of the ingredients together and apply to the greasy parts of your head. Leave in place for about 5 minutes to allow the excess oil to be completely absorbed and then brush out. If you are finding that the hair is dry and static as a result of this treatment, spray hair spray on your brush and brush the underside of the hair with it - this should help you to tame strays.

Chapter 9:

How to Choose the Right Oils Every Time

Getting this Right is Vital to Success

When it comes to choosing the essential oil that is best for your condition, the choice is more complicated than simply choosing the oil with the right properties.

When choosing an oil you also need to consider how easy it is to blend, how it will be applied, when it will be applied and whether or not you like the smell.

Take Tea Tree oil as an example. It has a very strong scent and does not blend well with too many other oils. I personally really do not like the smell and so I avoid using it, even though it is a very potent oil.

If you have a cold or flu, its strong anti-bacterial and anti-viral properties could come in handy.

Looking for Oils That Play Well With Others

Essential oils are very potent and blending synergistic oils can make them even more so. You can create a much more effective treatment by blending two or more oils together.

Some oils, such as Lavender oil, blend easily with others. Others, such as Tea Tree oil, do not blend that well with many other oils. If you need to choose between two oils to keep in your kit, I would advise choosing the oil that is easier to blend. This will allow you to make a much wider variety of blends in future.

You will learn more about how to blend oils in Chapter 4.

How the Oil Will Be Applied

This is where the actual consistency of the oil can come into play. The name, essential oils, is actually a bit of a misnomer as these compounds are not actually oils at all but more the essence of the plant.

There are two things to consider when you are deciding how you will use the oil - the method of application, whether it is through massage, diffusion, etc. and the consistency of the oil itself.

Determining how you will use the oil beforehand is essential. Lemon Grass oil, for example, can be quite useful in treating colds and flu. You have to be careful though as it can irritate the skin. In this instance, it would be better to diffuse the oil.

If, however, you have sore and tight shoulders, a blend that you can rub in or add to the bath would be a lot more useful and you would need to choose an oil, like Marjoram oil.

The actual viscosity of the oil may also come into play - some oils, such as Benzoin, are more resinous in nature and thus will not flow as well as the others. This could make blending more of a challenge.

When You Will Apply the Oils

When you are going to apply the oils is also important. You need to remember that the oils act not only on the physical body but also on the mind. Using Rosemary oil, for example, in a blend for sore muscles can be very helpful - but not if you are going to apply it in the hours leading up to bedtime. Rosemary oil is a powerful mental stimulant and you are likely to have trouble sleeping.

Citrus oils, for example, can cause your skin to become more photo-sensitive so it is not a good idea to apply these before going out into the sun.

Whether or Not You Like the Smell

My mother used to tell me that the worse I thought my medicine tasted, the better it actually was for me. In aromatherapy, the opposite is true.

Whilst the properties of the oil are not affected by whether or not you like its smell, its overall efficacy is. It's simple - the better you like the smell, the better your mind will respond to it.

I, for example, do not like the smell of lavender essential oil. Despite the fact that it is one of the most soothing oils, if I put a few drops on my pillow, I quickly get annoyed with the smell and have to swap the pillow out. For me personally, Sandalwood is a much better bet to enable me to drift off to sleep.

Your own preferences will be different so I advise you to play around with the different groups of scents to narrow down the scents that you like best. Perhaps you prefer the fresh smell of citrus oils, or perhaps you prefer the scent of the floral oils. Your personal preferences are worth determining if you are to find the perfect oil for you.

Chapter 10:
Quick Reference

Skin Complaints

Acne: Bergamot, cedarwood chamomile, clary sage, clove bud, galbanum, geranium, grapefruit, helichrysum, juniper, lavandin, lavender, lemon, lemongrass, lime,, mandarin, myrtle, niaouli, palmarosa, peppermint, patchouli, petitgrain, rosemary, rosewood, spearmint, sandalwood, tea tree, thyme, vetiver, yarrow, ylang ylang.

Allergies: Chamomile, helichrysum, lemon balm, true lavender.

Athlete's foot: Clove bud, eucalyptus, lavender, lemon, lemongrass, myrrh, patchouli, tea tree.

Baldness & hair care: Bay leaf, birch, cedarwood, chamomile, grapefruit, juniper, patchouli, rosemary, sage, yarrow, ylang ylang.

Boils, abscesses & blisters: Bergamot, chamomile, clary sage, eucalyptus, galbanum, helichrysum, lavender, lemon, mastic, niaouli, tea tree, thyme.

Bruises: Arnica (use as a lotion, not neat), clove bud, dill, fennel, geranium, hyssop, sweet marjoram, lavender, thyme.

Burns: Balsam, chamomile, clove bud, eucalyptus, geranium, helichrysum, lavender marigold, niaouli, tea tree, yarrow.

Chapped & cracked skin: Balsam, benzoin, myrrh, patchouli, sandalwood.

Chilblains: Black pepper, chamomile, lemon, lime, sweet marjoram.

Cold sores/herpes simplex: Bergamot, eucalyptus, lemon, tea tree.

Congested & dull skin: Angelica, birch, sweet fennel, geranium, grapefruit, lavender, lemon, lime, mandarin, myrtle, neroli, niaouli, orange, palmarosa, peppermint, rose, rosemary, rosewood, spearmint, ylang ylang.

Cuts/sores: Balsam, benzoin, borneol, chamomile, clove bud, eucalyptus, galbanum, geranium, helichrysum, hyssop, lavender, lemon, lime, linaloe, marigold, mastic, myrrh, niaouli, pine, sage, tea tree, thyme, vetiver, and yarrow.

Dandruff: Bay leaf, cade, cedarwood, eucalyptus, lavender, lemon, patchouli, rosemary, sage, tea tree.

Dermatitis: Birch, cade, cananga, carrot seed, cedarwood, chamomile, geranium, helichrysum, hops, hyssop, juniper, true lavender, palmarosa, patchouli, peppermint, rosemary, sage spearmint, thyme.

Dry & sensitive skin: Balsam, cassie, chamomile, frankincense, jasmine, lavandin, lavender, rosewood, sandalwood.

Eczema: Balsam, bergamot, cade, carrot seed, cedarwood, chamomile, geranium, helichrysum, hyssop, juniper, lavandin, lavender, lemon balm, marigold, myrrh, patchouli, rose rosemary, sage, thyme, violet, yarrow.

Excessive perspiration: Citronella, cypress, lemongrass, petitgrain, pine, sage.

Greasy or oily skin/scalp: Bay leaf, bergamot, cajeput, cananga, carrot seed, citronella, cypress, sweet fennel, geranium, jasmine, juniper, lavender, lemon, lemongrass, litsea cubeba, mandarin, marigold, mimosa, myrtle, niaouli, palmarosa, patchouli, petitgrain, rosemary, rosewood, sandalwood, clary sage, tea tree, thyme, vetiver, ylang ylang.

Hemorrhoids/piles: Balsam, coriander, cubebs, cypress, geranium, juniper, myrrh, myrtle, parsley, yarrow.

Insect bites: Lemon balm, basil, bergamot, cajeput, cananga, chamomile, cinnamon leaf, eucalyptus, lavandin, lavender, lemon, marigold, niaouli, tea tree, thyme, ylang ylang.

Insect repellent: Lemon balm, basil, bergamot, borneol, cedarwood, citronella, clove bud, cypress, eucalyptus, geranium, lavender, lemongrass, litsea cubeba, mastic, patchouli, rosemary.

Irritated & inflamed skin: Angelica, benzoin, cedarwood, chamomile, elemi, helichrysum, hyssop, jasmine, lavandin, true lavender, marigold, myrrh, patchouli, rose, clary sage, spikenard, tea tree, yarrow.

Lice: Cinnamon leaf, eucalyptus, galbanum, geranium, lavandin, lavender, parsley, pine, rosemary, thyme.

Mouth & gum infections/ulcers: Bergamot, cypress, sweet fennel, lemon, mastic, myrrh, orange, sage, thyme.

Psoriasis: Angelica, bergamot, birch, carrot seed, chamomile, true lavender.

Rashes: Balsam, carrot seed, chamomile, hops, true lavender, marigold, sandalwood, spikenard, tea tree, yarrow.

Ringworm: Geranium, spike lavender, mastic, mint (peppermint & spearmint), myrrh, Levant styrax, tea tree.

Scabies: Balsam, bergamot, cinnamon leaf, lavandin, lavender, lemongrass, mastic, peppermint, pine, rosemary, Levant styrax, spearmint, thyme.

Scars & stretch marks: Cabreuva, elemi, frankincense, galbanum, true lavender, mandarin, orange blossom, palmarosa, patchouli, rosewood, sandalwood, spikenard, violet, yarrow.

Slack tissue: Geranium, grapefruit, juniper, lemongrass, lime, mandarin, sweet marjoram, neroli, black pepper, petitgrain, rosemary, yarrow.

Spots: Bergamot, cade, cajeput, eucalyptus, helichrysum, lavender, lemon, lime, litsea cubeba, mandarin, niaouli, tea tree.

Ticks: Sweet marjoram.

Toothache & teething pain: Chamomile, clove bud, mastic, mint, myrrh, peppermint, spearmint.

Varicose veins: Cypress, lemon, lime, orange blossom, yarrow.

Verrucae: Tea tree.

Warts & corns: Cinnamon leaf, lemon, lime, tea tree.

Wounds: Canadian balsam, Peru balsam, Tolu balsam, bergamot, cabreuva, chamomile, clove bud, cypress, elemi, eucalyptus, frankincense, galbanum, geranium, helichrysum, hyssop, juniper, lavandin, lavender, linaloe, marigold, mastic, myrrh, niaouli, patchouli, rosewood, Levant styrax, tea tree, vetiver, yarrow.

Wrinkles & mature skin: Carrot seed, elemi, sweet fennel, frankincense, galbanum, geranium, jasmine, labdanum, true lavender, mandarin, mimosa, myrrh, orange blossom, palmarosa, patchouli, rose, rosewood, clary sage, sandalwood, spikenard, ylang ylang.

Circulation, Muscles and Joints

Accumulation of toxins: Angelica, birch, carrot seed, celery seed, coriander, cumin, sweet fennel, grapefruit, juniper, lovage, parsley.

Aches and pains: Ambrette, star anise, aniseed, basil, bay leaf, cajeput, calamintha, chamomile, coriander, eucalyptus, galbanum, ginger, helichrysum, lavandin, lavender, lemongrass, sweet marjoram, mastic, mint (peppermint & spearmint), niaouli, nutmeg, black pepper, pine, rosemary, sage, thyme, turmeric, vetiver.

Arthritis: Allspice, angelica, benzoin, birch, cajeput, carrot seed, cedarwood , celery seed, chamomile, clove bud, coriander, eucalyptus (blue gum & peppermint), silver fir, ginger, guaiac wood, juniper, lemon, sweet marjoram, mastic, myrrh, nutmeg, parsley, black pepper, pine, rosemary, sage, thyme, turmeric, vetiver, yarrow.

Cellulitis: Birch, cypress, sweet fennel, geranium, grapefruit, juniper, lemon, parsley, rosemary, thyme.

Debility/poor muscle tone: Allspice, ambrette, borneol, ginger, grapefruit, sweet marjoram, black pepper, pine, rosemary, sage.

Edema & water retention: Angelica, birch, carrot seed, cypress, sweet fennel, geranium, grapefruit, juniper, lovage, mandarin, orange, rosemary, sage.

Gout: Angelica, French basil, benzoin, carrot seed, celery seed, coriander, guaiac wood, juniper, lovage, mastic, pine, rosemary, thyme.

High blood pressure & hypertension: Lemon balm, cananga, true lavender, lemon, sweet marjoram, clary sage, yarrow, ylang ylang.

Muscular cramp & stiffness: Allspice, ambrette, coriander, cypress, grapefruit, jasmine, lavandin, lavender, sweet marjoram, black pepper, pine, rosemary, thyme, vetiver.

Obesity: White birch, sweet fennel, juniper, lemon, mandarin, orange.

Palpitations: Orange, orange blossom, rose, ylang ylang.

Poor circulation & low blood pressure: Ambrette, balsam, bay leaf, benzoin, white birch, borneol, cinnamon leaf, coriander, cumin, cypress, eucalyptus blue gum, galbanum, geranium, ginger, lemon, lemongrass, lovage, niaouli, nutmeg, orange blossom, black pepper, pine, rose, rosemary, sage, thyme, violet.

Rheumatism: Allspice, angelica, star anise, aniseed, balsam, basil, bay leaf, benzoin, white birch, borneol, cajeput, calamintha, carrot seed, cedarwood, celery seed, chamomile, cinnamon leaf, clove bud, coriander, cypress, eucalyptus, sweet fennel, silver fir, galbanum, ginger, helichrysum, juniper, lavandin, lavender, lemon, lovage, sweet marjoram, mastic, niaouli, nutmeg, parsley, black pepper, pine, rosemary, Spanish sage, thyme, turmeric, vetiver, violet, yarrow.

Sprains & strains: Bay leaf, borneol, chamomile, clove bud, eucalyptus, ginger, helichrysum, jasmine, lavandin, lavender, sweet marjoram, black pepper, pine , rosemary, thyme, turmeric, vetiver.

Respiratory System

Asthma: Asafetida, lemon balm, Canadian balsam, Peru balsam, benzoin, cajeput, clove bud, costus, cypress, elecampane, eucalyptus, frankincense, galbanum, helichrysum, hops, hyssop, lavandin, lavender, lemon, lime, sweet marjoram, mint, myrrh, myrtle, niaouli, pine, rose, rosemary, sage, tea tree, thyme.

Bronchitis: Angelica, star anise, aniseed, asafetida, lemon balm, balsam, copaiba balsam, basil, benzoin, borneol, cajeput, caraway, cascarilla bark, cedarwood, clove bud, costus, cypress, elecampane, elemi, eucalyptus, frankincense, galbanum, helichrysum, hyssop, labdanum, lavandin, lavender, lemon, sweet marjoram, mastic, peppermint & spearmint, myrrh, myrtle, niaouli, orange, pine, rosemary, sandalwood, hemlock spruce, tea tree, thyme, violet.

Catarrh: Balsam, cajeput, cedar wood, elecampane, elemi, eucalyptus, frankincense, galbanum, ginger, hyssop, jasmine, lavandin, lavender, lemon, lime, mastic, peppermint & spearmint, myrrh, myrtle, niaouli, black pepper, pine, sandalwood, Levant styrax, tea tree, thyme, violet.

Chill: Balsam, benzoin, cabreuva, calamintha, cinnamon leaf, ginger, grapefruit, orange, black pepper.

Chronic coughs: Lemon balm, balsam, costus, cubebs, cypress, elecampane, elemi, frankincense, galbanum, helichrysum, hops, hyssop, jasmine, peppermint & spearmint, myrrh, myrtle, sandalwood, Levant styrax.

Coughs: Angelica, star anise, aniseed, balsam, basil, benzoin, borneol, cabreuva, cajeput, caraway, cascarilla bark, cedarwood, eucalyptus, ginger, hyssop, labdanum, sweet marjoram, myrrh, niaouli, black pepper, pine, rose, rosemary, sage, tea tree.

Croup: Balsam.

Earache: Basil, chamomile, lavender.

Halitosis/offensive breath: Bergamot, cardamom, sweet fennel, lavandin, lavender, peppermint & spearmint, myrrh.

Laryngitis/hoarseness: Balsam, benzoin, caraway, cubebs, lemon eucalyptus, frankincense, jasmine, lavandin, lavender, myrrh, sage, sandalwood, thyme.

Sinusitis: Basil, cajeput, cubebs, eucalyptus blue gum, ginger, labdanum, peppermint, niaouli, pine, tea tree.

Sore throat & throat infections: Balsam, bergamot, cajeput, eucalyptus, geranium, ginger, hyssop, lavandin, lavender, myrrh, myrtle, niaouli, pine, sage, sandalwood, tea tree, thyme, violet.

Tonsillitis: Bergamot, geranium, hyssop, myrtle, sage, thyme.

Whooping cough: Asafetida, helichrysum, hyssop, true lavender, mastic, niaouli, rosemary, sage, tea tree.

Digestive System

Colic: Star anise, aniseed, lemon balm, calamintha, caraway, cardamom, carrot seed, chamomile, clove bud, coriander, cumin, dill, sweet fennel, ginger, hyssop, lavandin, lavender, sweet marjoram, peppermint & spearmint, neroli, parsley, black pepper, rosemary, clary sage.

Constipation & sluggish digestion: Cinnamon leaf, cubebs, sweet fennel, lovage, sweet marjoram, nutmeg, orange, palmarosa, black pepper, tarragon, turmeric, yarrow.

Cramp/gastric spasm: Allspice, star anise, aniseed, caraway, cardamom, cinnamon leaf, coriander, costus, cumin, galbanum, ginger, lavandin, lavender, lovage, peppermint & spearmint, orange, neroli, black pepper, clary sage, lemon verbena, yarrow.

Griping pains: Cardoon, dill, sweet fennel, parsley.

Heartburn: Cardoon, black pepper.

Indigestion/flatulence: Allspice, angelica, star anise, aniseed, lemon balm, basil, calamintha, caraway, cardamom, carrot seed, cascarilla bark, celery seed, chamomile, cinnamon leaf, clove bud, coriander, costus, cubebs, cumin, dill, sweet fennel, galbanum, ginger, hops, hyssop, lavandin, lavender, lemongrass, linden, litsea cubeba, lovage, mandarin, sweet marjoram, peppermint & spearmint, myrrh, nutmeg, orange, neroli, parsley, black pepper, petitgrain, rosemary, clary sage, thyme, valerian, lemon verbena, yarrow.

Liver congestion: Carrot seed, celery seed, helichrysum, linden, rose, rosemary, sage, turmeric, lemon verbena.

Loss of appetite: Bergamot, caraway, cardamom, ginger, myrrh, black pepper.

Nausea/vomiting: Allspice, lemon balm, French basil, cardamom, cascarilla bark, chamomile, clove bud, coriander, sweet fennel, ginger, lavandin, lavender, peppermint & spearmint, nutmeg, black pepper, rose, rosewood, sandalwood.

Genitourinary and Endocrine Systems

Amenorrhea/lack of menstruation: Basil, carrot seed, celery seed, cinnamon leaf, dill, sweet fennel, hops, hyssop, juniper, lovage, sweet marjoram, myrrh, parsley, rose, sage, yarrow.

Dysmenorrhea/cramp, painful or difficult menstruation: Lemon balm, basil, carrot seed, chamomile, cypress, frankincense, hops, jasmine, juniper, lavandin, lavender, lovage, sweet marjoram, rose, rosemary, sage, yarrow.

Cystitis: Balsam, bergamot, cedarwood, celery seed, chamomile, cubebs, eucalyptus blue gum, frankincense, juniper, lavandin, lavender, lovage, mastic, niaouli, parsley, Scotch pine, sandalwood, tea tree, thyme, yarrow.

Frigidity: Cassie, cinnamon leaf, jasmine, nutmeg, orange blossom, parsley, patchouli, black pepper, cabbage rose, rosewood, clary sage, sandalwood, ylang ylang.

Lack of nursing milk: Celery seed, dill, sweet fennel, hops.

Labor pain & childbirth aid: Cinnamon leaf, jasmine, true lavender, nutmeg, parsley, rose, clary sage.

Leucorrhoea/white discharge from the vagina: Bergamot, cedarwood, cinnamon leaf, cubebs, eucalyptus blue gum, frankincense, hyssop, lavandin, lavender, sweet marjoram, mastic, myrrh, rosemary, clary sage, sandalwood, tea tree.

Menopausal problems: Cypress, sweet fennel, geranium, jasmine, rose.

Menorrhagia/excessive menstruation: Chamomile, cypress, rose.

Premenstrual tension /PMT: Carrot seed, chamomile, geranium, true lavender, sweet marjoram, neroli.

Pruritis/itching: Bergamot, Atlas cedarwood, juniper, lavender, myrrh, tea tree.

Sexual over activity: Hops, sweet marjoram.

Thrush/candida: Bergamot, geranium, myrrh, tea tree.

Urethritis: Bergamot, cubebs, mastic, tea tree.

Immune System

Chickenpox: Bergamot, chamomile, eucalyptus, true lavender, tea tree.

Colds/Flu: Angelica, star anise, aniseed, balsam, basil, bergamot, borneol, cabreuva, cajeput, caraway, cinnamon leaf, citronella, clove bud, coriander, eucalyptus, frankincense, ginger, grapefruit, helichrysum, juniper, lemon, lime, sweet marjoram, mastic, peppermint & spearmint, myrtle, niaouli, orange, pine, rosemary, rosewood, sage, tea tree, thyme, yarrow.

Fever: Basil, bergamot, borneol, eucalyptus, ginger, helichrysum, juniper, lemon, lemongrass, lime, peppermint & spearmint, myrtle, niaouli, rosemary, rosewood, sage, tea tree, thyme, yarrow.

Measles: Bergamot, eucalyptus blue gum, lavender, tea tree.

Nervous System

Allergies: Chamomile, helichrysum, lemon balm, true lavender.

Anxiety: Ambrette, lemon balm, French basil, bergamot, cananga, frankincense, hyssop, jasmine, juniper, true lavender, mimosa, neroli, Levant styrax, lemon verbena, ylang ylang.

Depression: Allspice, ambrette, lemon balm, balsam, basil, bergamot, cassie, grapefruit, helichrysum, jasmine, true lavender, neroli, rose, clary sage, sandalwood, vetiver, ylang ylang.

Headache: Chamomile, citronella, cumin, eucalyptus, grapefruit, hops, lavandin, lavender, lemongrass, linden, sweet marjoram, peppermint & spearmint, rose, rosemary, rosewood, sage, thyme, violet.

Insomnia: Lemon balm, basil, calamintha, chamomile, hops, true lavender, linden, mandarin, sweet marjoram, neroli, petitgrain, rose, sandalwood, thyme, valerian, lemon verbena, vetiver, violet, yarrow, ylang ylang.

Migraine: Angelica, lemon balm, basil, chamomile, citronella, coriander, true lavender, linden, sweet marjoram, peppermint & spearmint, clary sage, valerian, yarrow.

Nervous exhaustion or fatigue/debility: Allspice, angelica, asafetida, basil, borneol, cardamom, cassie, cinnamon leaf, citronella, coriander, costus, cumin, elemi, eucalyptus, ginger, grapefruit, helichrysum, hyacinth, hyssop, jasmine, lavandin, spike lavender, lemongrass, peppermint & spearmint, nutmeg, palmarosa, patchouli, petitgrain, pine, rosemary, sage, thyme, vetiver, violet, ylang ylang.

Neuralgia/sciatica: Allspice, borneol, celery seed, chamomile, citronella, coriander, eucalyptus, geranium, helichrysum, hops, spike lavender, sweet marjoram, mastic, peppermint & spearmint, nutmeg, pine, rosemary.

Nervous tension and stress: Allspice, ambrette, angelica, asafetida, lemon balm, balsam, basil, benzoin, bergamot, borneol, calamintha, cananga, cardamom, cassie, cedarwood, chamomile, cinnamon leaf, costus, cypress, elemi, frankincense, galbanum, geranium, helichrysum, hops, hyacinth, hyssop, jasmine, juniper, true lavender, lemongrass, linaloe, linden, mandarin, sweet marjoram, mimosa, peppermint & spearmint, orange, neroli, palmarosa, patchouli, petitgrain, pine, rose, rosemary, rosewood, clary sage, sandalwood, thyme, valerian, lemon verbena, vetiver, violet, yarrow, ylang ylang.

Shock: Lemon balm, lavandin, lavender, neroli.

Vertigo: Lemon balm, lavandin, lavender, peppermint & spearmint

Chapter 11:
The Top Oils to Consider

Oils That Should Be On Your Shopping List

When it comes to which oils to choose, you will be guided by your own personal preference. The oils on this list are the ones that I have found to be most useful and that I find that I use most of all.

As you get to know the characters of the oils, you will instinctively begin to know which oils mix with which others for best results.

All I can say for now is that you should choose a few of the oils on this list - if possible try to smell testers before making your buying decision. Then go out and get the best quality of the oils that you like that you are able to afford.

Please note that these are some of my favorite oils but it is not a list that is set in stone for you, only those I recommend for beginners unsure of what to start with.

You need to find oils that suit your own tastes – If, for example, you prefer less exotic scents, maybe switch out ylang ylang for geranium oil.

Whatever you choose, as long as you go with something that you really love, you will always find a use for it.

Eucalyptus

If you don't have this in your first aid kit, you are missing out. There really is no oil that is better for freshening up a sick room and helping to unblock a blocked nose. Mix some eucalyptus and tea tree oils and diffuse them in the room as a major weapon against all sorts of bugs.

Alternatively, mix some into an aqueous base and rub onto the back and chest to clear a tight chest. Rub the same mix into your feet at night, just before bed and you will feel a whole lot better in the morning.

Eucalyptus is also great for treating sore and tired muscles. Mix into an oil base and apply to sore muscles or put some drops in the bath or a foot bath.

The smell is quite strong but not quite as overpowering as is the case with Tea Tree oil and I find that it is a much better decongestant anyway. It can be hard to blend eucalyptus because of its fragrance but I have found that lime oil or lemon oil and eucalyptus oil blend particularly well together and provide a potent anti-bacterial mixture, perfect for the sick room or for disinfecting kitchen surfaces.

Sandalwood

I love sandalwood, I love the smell, I love the effect on my skin and I love how relaxing it is. If I am battling to sleep at night, a few drops on my pillow soon has me off to dreamland.

Sandalwood is a great healer when it comes to stress and tension and it is deeply relaxing. Use in a diffuser or make up a blend. Sandalwood blends really well with lavender and vetiver for complete relaxation. It is also great blended with neroli for when you are feeling stressed out.

For the skin, it is good for drier, mature skin that needs a bit of love and care. Mixed with neroli and rose hip oil it makes a fantastic moisturizing treatment.

Sandalwood is a wonderful base note and acts as a fixative in blends.

Neroli

Again, one of my favorites - this oil can lift your spirits at any time and smells really good in blends. It goes with most other oils so you will not often be without a partner for it.

Use when you are feeling really upset or anxious, or when you are feeling really depressed. Diffuse it into the atmosphere but do be warned not to use it in too small a space - a friend and eye used it in the car one day and ended up what seemed close to being high.

Neroli is also wonderful on the skin and can help to banish stretch marks and scars. Apply every day, twice a day - you choose the base to use. My favorite for scars is a sweet almond oil base with some rose hip oil added in.

Benzoin

Benzoin doesn't blend as well as some of the others but it really is worth keeping a spot for. It is one of the best oils to help deal with depression and stress and makes you feel euphoric, especially if you use it with jasmine.

I prefer to use benzoin in a burner - I add in a few drops of neroli, a few drops of benzoin and either sandalwood or cedarwood and it is a blend that allows me to push through stressful deadlines feeling completely relaxed and rested.

It is one of the less viscous oils so using it can be a bit of a pain - what I will normally do is to pull out the dropper section and dip a skewer into the oil to get it out faster. If you do not do this on a cold day it might not even come out of the dropper at all.

Benzoin smells a lot like vanilla and so it is one of the best oils to add to a milk and honey bath if you do not want something with a plainer fragrance.

Jasmine

I do use a blend when it comes to Jasmine oil but it is one of the better brands. The extra expense is well worth it. Jasmine is another of those oils that mix with just about every other oil and it is wonderful to have in first aid kit. It helps create a feeling of happiness and will lift your spirits.

The smell of jasmine might be a bit overpowering - if you find that this is the case, do not give up - blend it with other oils and see what an amazing note it lends to the blend. It can soften harsher notes easily. Jasmine is a good oil to have if you want to play around with making your own perfume.

Rose

Again, I use a good quality blend - the absolute would just be too expensive. Like jasmine, it mixes with just about any other essential oil and lends a deep, exotic fragrance to the blend. For perfumes there truly is no more heavenly mix than rose oil, with jasmine oil, neroli oil, sandalwood oil and a touch of ylang ylang oil.

Rose is good for skin ailments - burns, rashes, etc. and has excellent regenerative properties. It is good for helping you deal with stress and depression and helps to boost spirits as well.

Lavender

Lavender oil has a clean, herbaceous scent and is one of the most versatile oils to have, especially if you have kids. The oil is gentle enough to be used on children from the age of 10 weeks and is wonderfully calming and healing and most children do like the smell.

I am pretty sure that this is the oil that you will use most often so I advise that you make up a blend, diluted according to the rules in Chapter 3, to keep ready when necessary.

Many books advise applying Lavender oil neat to skin but I don't agree with this. It is okay to do so on occasion when your kids get a little older but, as a general rule, I would dilute the oil first. It is just as effective diluted.

Apply to scratches, minor burns and skin rashes. Rub on sore tummies and into the temples when your child has a headache. If your child is upset or over-tired, Lavender oil can be wonderfully calming. I often found that I could distract my kids when a temper tantrum was threatening by getting out the Lavender blend getting them to rub it into their palms, just as you would a hand cream. The kids find the action soothing and it can distract them long enough to make them forget about the tantrum. (It doesn't always work though.)

Lavender diffused in your child's room will help them to have a peaceful and quiet night's rest. It can help treat allergic reactions and reduce the symptoms of pain and fever.

For older children, Lavender can be useful in the treatment of acne and for helping out with exam stress and muscular aches and pains.

If there is only one oil that you can get, this is it.

Lavender oil, combined with Chamomile oil is one of the most useful, synergistic blends that a parent can have.

Chamomile

It is amazing to me how the humble little Chamomile flower can produce such a potent remedy. I still use it in place of Clove oil when I have a toothache and find that it works as well, if not better.

Chamomile is definitely second on the list of oils that you have to have. It is also gentle enough to be used from ages 10 weeks and up and is a great companion to Lavender oil.

Blend it into an organic aqueous base and you have a soothing, multi-purpose cream that will help fight inflammation and allergic skin conditions. Apply to soothe diaper rash and dry, sensitive skin. Mixing it with Sandalwood or Cedar Wood anchors it and improves the skin soothing action of the oil.

It can also alleviate the pain associated with sunburn and minor burns and help to stimulate the regeneration of damaged skin. Apply in the form of a cold compress as soon as the child burns themselves and it can help to reduce blistering as well.

In a warm compress it can help alleviate pain and fever - it is especially useful when it comes to earache and toothache. It is one of the oils with the strongest analgesic properties.

It blends well with Lavender and Sandalwood oil for a really calming base to soothe even the most frazzled nerves - useful for both teenagers and the parents of teenagers.

Tea Tree

Tea Tree always smells so medicinal to me so I would never use it in a blend for relaxing or stress. There are some people who like its strong scent though and so they find it useful to blend. It does smell better when mixed with Eucalyptus. It is a potent antibacterial, antiviral and anti-fungal agent.

This is one of those few times when I suggest using an oil neat - when there is a fungal infection like Ringworm, apply the oil neat three to four times a day and continue to apply twice a day for at least another week once the fungal infection has cleared up to prevent reinfection.

The oil can be diffused or added to the bath water to chase away the flu virus. Mixed with Eucalyptus oil and a suitable carrier oil, you can use it as a foot rub to help treat colds and the flu and to reduce fevers.

Added to the water used to clean the floors and wipe down the counters, it becomes a valuable natural and anti-bacterial cleaner and will allow you to do away with harsh cleaning chemicals that could be harming the health of your kids.

A blend of Tea Tree oil and Lavender oil in the appropriate amount of carrier oil can be applied to clear up infected sinuses. Using Tea Tree oil, Eucalyptus oil and Lavender oil can in a diffuser will help clear up congestion and prevent the spread of infection.

This is another oil with multiple uses and it has been proven to be as effective as conventional bactericidal agents.

That said, it is not an oil that is easy to blend with others and so you may find that you will use it mainly on its own. For this reason, and because of the strong smell, you may decide to leave this until last when collecting your oils.

Ylang Ylang

Ylang ylang is another really exotic oil. You will either love it or you will hate it. This is a great oil to have around if you want to relax and it has aphrodisiac qualities if you have loving on the mind.

Ylang ylang can be blended with neroli and sandalwood to give you a blend that will help you deal with whatever stress you are under.

As it has quite a strong scent, add it last and only one drop at a time. Mixed with sandalwood - double the am out of sandalwood to the amount of ylang ylang, it ensures a peaceful night's sleep.

I do advise skipping the ylang ylang if you have a bit of a headache, the strong smell can make it worse.

Geranium

This has a fairly strong scent and, to me at least, smells more like an herb than a floral scent. It is, however, classified as a floral note and is often used as a replacement for Rose oil in blends.

This is one of the more gentle oils and is extremely useful when it comes to dealing with issues relating to the skin. Geranium oil must be diluted before use but is great when mixed with Lavender oil to treat scratches and allergic skin reactions.

It is also a great skin regenerator and so is useful in the treatment of scars and burns.

On a mental level, Geranium helps you to relax and can also help your children to sleep. It is an uplifting oil as well and can be useful in the treatment of depression.

Bergamot

Bergamot is one of the citrus oils but does not have a distinctly citrus scent. It blends quite well with other oils and is really great for use when it comes to treating troubled, oily skin conditions and is valuable in the treatment of acne. Care should be taken as the oil is photo-toxic - it should never be applied just before going out into the sun.

This is one of the best oils for treating depression and combating stress. It will help to treat insomnia that is brought on by stress.

It does have antibacterial properties as well and can be used as an effective remedy for colds and the flu.

If insects are pestering your children, add a few drops of Bergamot to the bath water or into a cream base with a few drops of Lavender for an effective insect repellent.

Vertiver

Vertiver oil is also known as the oil of tranquility and has a very deep and lingering scent and provides a good base for other blends. It is an oil that promotes deep relaxation and that is very useful when diffused for treating the symptoms of stress and insomnia.

It is also very valuable when it comes to easing sore and tired muscles - use in a blend with Sandalwood oil for sprains and strains or muscles that are overworked. It is also very effective for relieving muscular aches brought on by stress and tension.

This oil is quite thick but a little goes a long way so it is worth including in this list. It can overpower other oils in the blend easily so only add in one drop at a time.

Chapter 12:

Oils That You Should <u>Never</u> Buy

These Should Never Make it into Your Home

The list of oils that <u>should not</u> be used is notably shorter than the useful list but there are some oils on this list that I have seen in recipes for a lot of different body scrubs. Whilst it is true that these oils do have some useful qualities, they have components in them that make them undesirable for other reasons.

As a general rule, if you find an oil that you have never heard of before or you find an oil from a plant that you know is a noxious weed or one that is inedible, it is best to do further research before you do buy it.

Cinnamon oil

This is a tough one, especially around the holidays but Cinnamon simply does not have enough uses to really recommend it for use in the home. You could, if you really wanted to, use it as a fragrance oil but never use the essential oil on your skin. It is highly irritating to the skin and has compounds that are difficult for the body to process. It is also very dangerous for pets.

Clove oil

This is not such a hard one to avoid but if you must use Clove oil, make sure that it is the Clove Bud oil. The rest are too high in toxins to be used. This oil can also really irritate the skin and can be toxic to pets.

Rosewood oil

Rosewood oil is actually a very good oil to use - it is nourishing and great for dry skin. Why is it on this list then? The Rosewood tree is endangered and the oil cannot be produced without causing some damage to the tree.

Tansy or Rue oils

You are not likely to be able to find these easily but both are highly toxic and should be completely avoided.

Conclusion

Thank you again for downloading this book!

I hope that you have learned a lot about aromatherapy and how to use it in your day to day life. I also hope that you will treat this book as a stepping stone on the path to learning more about the amazing world of aromatherapy.

All that is left is for you to go out and explore this exciting hobby on your own - be warned, once the bug has bitten, you will never give it up! If you feel like you need some more guidance, take a look at some of my other titles available on Amazon.

Lastly, I would really like to ask a favor of you – Please take the time to share your thoughts and post a review on Amazon. Feedback is very important for self-published authors such as myself.

Thank you and good luck!

www.ingramcontent.com/pod-product-compliance
Lightning Source LLC
Chambersburg PA
CBHW062042280526
45788CB00003B/1075